Endomorph Diet for Men

A Beginner's 5-Week Step-by-Step Guide With Curated Recipes and a Meal Plan

mf

copyright © 2020 Tyler Spellmann

All rights reserved No part of this book may be reproduced, or stored in a retrieval system, or transmitted in any form or by any means, electronic, mechanical, photocopying, recording, or otherwise, without express written permission of the publisher.

Disclaimer

By reading this disclaimer, you are accepting the terms of the disclaimer in full. If you disagree with this disclaimer, please do not read the guide.

All of the content within this guide is provided for informational and educational purposes only, and should not be accepted as independent medical or other professional advice. The author is not a doctor, physician, nurse, mental health provider, or registered nutritionist/dietician. Therefore, using and reading this guide does not establish any form of a physician-patient relationship.

Always consult with a physician or another qualified health provider with any issues or questions you might have regarding any sort of medical condition. Do not ever disregard any qualified professional medical advice or delay seeking that advice because of anything you have read in this guide. The information in this guide is not intended to be any sort of medical advice and should not be used in lieu of any medical advice by a licensed and qualified medical professional.

The information in this guide has been compiled from a variety of known sources. However, the author cannot attest to or guarantee the accuracy of each source and thus should not be held liable for any errors or omissions.

You acknowledge that the publisher of this guide will not be held liable for any loss or damage of any kind incurred as a result of this guide or the reliance on any information provided within this guide. You acknowledge and agree that you assume all risk and responsibility for any action you undertake in response to the information in this guide.

Using this guide does not guarantee any particular result (e.g., weight loss or a cure). By reading this guide, you acknowledge that there are no guarantees to any specific outcome or results you can expect.

All product names, diet plans, or names used in this guide are for identification purposes only and are the property of their respective owners. The use of these names does not imply endorsement. All other trademarks cited herein are the property of their respective owners.

Where applicable, this guide is not intended to be a substitute for the original work of this diet plan and is, at most, a supplement to the original work for this diet plan and never a direct substitute. This guide is a personal expression of the facts of that diet plan.

Where applicable, persons shown in the cover images are stock photography models and the publisher has obtained the rights to use the images through license agreements with third-party stock image companies.

Table of Contents

Introduction — 6
Body Types — 8
  Ectomorph — 8
  Mesomorph — 9
  Endomorph — 9
Endomorph Body Type — 11
Endomorph Men — 14
  Bodybuilding — 14
  Sports — 15
  Cardio and Strength Training — 16
Endomorph Diet — 18
  Basic Endomorph Diet — 18
How to Follow an Endomorph Diet — 22
  Week 1: Identify Your Limits — 22
  Week 2: Replace Processed Food — 23
  Week 3: Reduce Carbs — 25
  Week 4: Devise a Weekly Plan — 28
  Week 5: Find Ways to Sustain — 33
Sample Recipes — 35
  Chicken Breast (Baked) — 36
  Grilled Chicken and Vegetables Skewers — 37
  Quinoa Salad with Avocado — 38
  Baked Salmon with Sweet Potato Fries — 39
  Turkey Meatballs with Spaghetti Squash — 40
  Chicken and Broccoli Stir-Fry — 41
  Beef and Vegetable Stew — 42
Conclusion — 43
FAQ and Quick Summary — 44
References and Helpful Links — 47

Introduction

Did you know that your genes can hinder you from getting that body goal you've always wanted?

Your genes hold a lot of valuable information to your physical attributes and if you want to change your body, you have to work with your natural body type.

The concept of somatotypes or body types was introduced in the 1940s by American psychologist William Herbert Sheldon. According to his research, there are three somatotypes: ectomorph, mesomorph, and endomorph. Each of these body types has its challenges and positives if one were to aim for an ideal body.

If you are wondering why a lot of popular diet fads and workout routines work for everyone else but you, remember that even in health and fitness, there is no such thing as a "one size fits all" solution. The best thing you can do is to learn how you can maximize what you have been given through your genes.

And a great way to start your journey to a better you is by knowing your body type. Are you an ectomorph, a mesomorph, or an endomorph?

Welcome to the Endomorph Diet for Men, a resource for all you need to know when it comes to endomorphs. This book is for men out there who are struggling with their endomorph body whether it be for weight loss, bodybuilding, or muscle gain.

In this guide, you will discover:

- What are the three somatotypes, their characteristics, and which one are you?
- What is an endomorph and how can you work with your body type?
- How should you eat based on your body type?
- What are the ways to follow your diet?
- Simple recipes you can incorporate into your meal plan

Body Types

William Herbert Sheldon, a researcher, and psychologist created three categories of body types or somatotypes based on body composition.

These types are (1) Ectomorph; (2) Mesomorph; and (3) Endomorph.

Ectomorph

When you think of ectomorphs, think of Lance Armstrong, Usain Bolt, Kevin Garnett, and Michael Phelps. Individuals with an ectomorph body type have lower body weight, are lean, and have long extremities. However, this does not mean that they have less body fat. They can be "skinny fat." Wherein, they are physically thin but with high body fat.

Men of this body type experience no difficulty in losing weight because of their accelerated metabolism. They have rapid energy expenditure. Hence, they can eat three buffets in a day and still keep their slim physique.

Although it seems to be a genetic advantage, this body type has a significant downside. Studies have shown that ectomorphs are more prone to nutrient deficiencies in the elderly. And have weaker bones and muscles. This is also why gaining muscle mass and visible body fat is a challenge to them.

They are better off following mild to moderate training with long intervals. Accompanied by a high protein diet.

Mesomorph

A mesomorph body type is usually seen in athletes who are well-built and muscular like Cristiano Ronaldo and Terrel Owens. They are seen with an "upright posture, long trunk, and short limbs." They have more muscle mass and fast-twitch muscle fibers, making it easier for them to engage in sports that require a lot of strength.

Individuals of this type experience no difficulty in losing or gaining weight—having a balance between body fat and muscle fat.

Endomorph

An endomorph; on the other hand, is usually seen in round body types.

Individuals with this body type gain weight faster than the other two types due to their slow metabolism. This is why physical activities should be part of their daily routine, as well as a more deliberate diet. More of this will be discussed in the following chapter.

Endomorph Body Type

An endomorph is described to have: (1) more fat cells; (2) a wider waist circumference relative to the chest; (3) a large head with a wide face; and (4) a stubby neck. Men have relatively less body fat than women which makes this body type more prominent in the female gender.

It may sound disheartening at first. But these characteristics do not need to be one's final features. Celebrities like Beyonce, Marilyn Monroe, Jennifer Lopez, and Scarlett Johansson are endomorphs who can use their curves to their advantage. A-listers like Chris Hemsworth, Chris Pratt, Dwayne Johnson, and Tom Hardy are all endomorphs who are known for their god-like physiques.

One can always choose to work towards an ideal endomorph body by possessing a strong will and discipline.

Take advantage of the fact that the endomorph body type has strong bones and is more capable of gaining muscle mass. With proper exercise and diet, a decrease in body fat content, and an increase in muscle growth can be achieved. Both are best done simultaneously because excessive estrogen production from uncontrolled fat deposition can slow down muscle growth.

Another challenge observed among endomorphs is a behavioral cycle. The sequence begins with gaining weight. Followed by low physical activity because of the difficulty of bearing one's weight. Consequently, eating more is due to a sedentary lifestyle.

With this behavior, combined with their genetically slower metabolism, they tend to convert excess calories into fat more easily.

Because of this, endomorphs are more susceptible to diabetes mellitus, hypertension, metabolic syndrome, and cancer.

This means that endomorphs need to put more effort into their daily routines. And be more intentional with what they consume.

A regular exercise routine should be followed to increase metabolism and reduce fat. A daily exercise should consist of cardiovascular workouts like running, swimming, or jogging for 30 to 60 minutes a day. And supplemented with strength training or high-intensity interval training (HIIT) two to three times a week to increase muscle mass. With muscle growth, more stored fat will be burned and more calories will be used even while resting.

Given the strong body structure of endomorphs, this should be maximized by doing a lot of bodyweight or weight-lifting exercises that require a lot of power.

And to continue burning calories during rest days, other forms of movement should still be part of the daily routine. If not for cardio exercises, walking or having bicycle rides should do the trick.

Endomorph Men

Men who identify as endomorphs or predominantly endomorph (if they are in combination with either ectomorph or mesomorph) are advantaged in many fields. As endomorphs are the strongest among body types, they do very well in fields where strength and a large physique is an advantage.

In this chapter, we will talk about bodybuilding and sports where endomorph men get a lot of recognition. We will also discuss a bit about cardio and strength training for endomorphs.

Bodybuilding

Men with Herculean frames are without a doubt the epitome of body aesthetics. Having an endomorph body is a strong point for bodybuilders as packing muscles comes easier for them than most hard gainers and makes them closer to the ideal bodybuilder image. What's more, they can maintain their muscles more easily, too, if they continue their training and remain on a calorie deficit diet.

The challenge of endomorph bodybuilders is that their body resists losing fat. This struggle is made more apparent during the cutting phase where they may lose more muscle mass than fat, and, hence, the duration of losing fat is longer than that of other body types.

For this, planning for long-term training and diet is a crucial part of the preparation for a competition or event. As for training, an endomorph bodybuilder's routine is filled with compound lifts be it bench presses, deadlifts, or squats. They can get a six-pack abs—that is if their abs are genetically structured to be so—when their body fat percentage dips to 10 percent or lower.

As for the diet, they tend to plan more carefully with their nutrition and strategize it together with their training. They are required to be more watchful in choosing their food and meal plans altogether. We will talk about more on this in the next chapter.

Some of the famous endomorph bodybuilders are Steve Davis, Lee Priest, and Dave Draper.

Sports

Endomorphs excel in strength sports, in general. Despite the challenge of stubborn body fats, this somatotype is prevalent in sports such as:

- football

- rugby
- shot put
- super-heavyweight boxing
- distance swimming
- wrestling, especially sumo wrestling
- discus and hammer throwing
- powerlifting

Think of athletes like NFL Vince Wilfork and Ndamukong Suh, and Icelandic powerlifter Benedikt Magnússon.

The challenge for endomorphs is though they may have strength, they must work harder for stamina or if they are carrying extra weight around for long periods of time. Thus, they may not do well with sports that require speed, agility, and endurance. However, this is just a predisposition and some endomorph athletes are able to succeed albeit with proper training and discipline.

Cardio and Strength Training

Cardio sports are rough for endomorphs though their large lung capacity makes them suitable for rowing. Workouts such as running may take a toll on their joints, but lower-impact cardio like biking, brisk walks, and long walks are good substitutes.

Endomorphs will need to incorporate daily cardio in their training to stay in a calorie deficit. Workouts such as a

30-minute elliptical or HIIT increase the metabolic rate when resting and training. This also improves aerobic and anaerobic pathways that strengthen respiration during a steady state of training. Cardio training also helps when training reaches plateaus.

Strength or resistance exercises such as circuit training are recommended for athletes, and for all endomorphs for health purposes, as these will involve short intense bouts of exercises with quick resting periods in between. It specifically helps in improving muscular fitness and may vary for individuals. Athletes train differently than bodybuilders, and powerlifters train differently than swimmers.

Lifting weights is not only great for muscle building but also for bones. Endomorphs are endowed with larger bones than their counterparts, to begin with. What lifting does is make the bones denser, tougher, and harder in response to the stress of the weights. Most weightlifting routines with lower repetition (6 reps or lower per set) are not great for burning calories and not as taxing for the respiratory system but advancing to moderate reps starts the activation.

The exercise requirements may be different for everyone. For beginners, more so when one is starting from a sedentary lifestyle or those with prior health conditions, it is wise to talk to a fitness coach first before embarking on any training.

Endomorph Diet

There are different techniques suggested for endomorphs. Some combine these techniques based on their lifestyle. Whereas, others simply follow the general endomorph diet.

Basic Endomorph Diet

For the basic endomorph diet, there is no calorie limit per day, but the macronutrients are divided into percentages.

30% for carbohydrates, 35% for protein, and 35% for fats.

An endomorph diet mostly consists of healthy fats, proteins, and complex carbohydrates.

To address the carbohydrate- and insulin-sensitivity of endomorphs, their diet should contain fewer carbohydrates and processed food. Coupled with an increase in protein intake to achieve muscle growth, break down fat, burn more calories, and reduce stored fat.

If you think you are not able to reach your protein goals from lean meat alone, you can add whey protein to your diet. Just make sure that you have no allergies to the ingredients and that you are cleared by your primary physician if you have a coexisting condition.

Sources of Protein and Mono- and Poly-Unsaturated Fats:

- Low-fat dairy products: Low-fat milk, yogurt, and cheese
- Poultry: Chicken and turkey
- Fish: Especially salmon, sardines, and tuna
- Non-tropical vegetable cooking oil: Olive, canola, and avocado oil
- Eggs and egg whites
- Non-tropical nuts: Almonds, hazelnuts, and walnuts

Sources of Carbohydrates:

- Dried beans, legumes, kidney beans, lentils, and chickpeas
- Fruits except for melons and pineapples
- Non-starchy vegetables: Broccoli, cauliflower, and celery
- Starchy vegetables: Sweet potatoes, yams, corn, and carrots
- Unrefined starchy vegetables: Quinoa and amaranth
- Whole-grain and whole-wheat products

Foods to Avoid:

- White bread and rice, pasta, and bagels
- Refined sweets and baked goods

- Soft drinks, energy drinks, and sports drinks
- Refined cereals, oatmeal, and puffed rice
- Processed and fried food
- Rich dairy products: Cream, whipped cream, and ice cream
- Red meat
- Sodium dense food
- Alcohol
- Cooking oils with saturated fat: Palm and coconut oil

You may combine the endomorph diet with the following methods to maximize weight loss:

Metabolic Confusion

In this method, you confuse your metabolism by alternating heavy calorie-days with fewer calorie-days. For example, you consume 2,000 calories today. Tomorrow, you consume 1,200 calories.

Another option would be a meal-to-meal basis. Wherein, you eat 600 calories for lunch and then 300 calories for dinner.

The theory behind this is that your metabolism will not create a fixed rate, but instead, will learn to adjust according to your food intake.

Carbohydrate Cycling

This technique tries to address the high carbohydrate sensitivity of endomorphs. It has the same idea as Metabolic Confusion, but just more focused on carbohydrates.

For example, you consume more carbohydrates on the days that you will be working out. (Preferably, not more than three days a week.) During your rest days, you eat fewer carbohydrates.

The advantages of this technique are:

- Your metabolism learns to adjust to varying amounts of caloric intake.
- Levels of insulin become more stable.
- Energy levels are distributed more evenly.
- Carbohydrate intake leads to muscle growth instead of fat restoration.
- Improves insulin sensitivity.

How to Follow an Endomorph Diet

Week 1: Identify Your Limits

Strategize your game plan by setting realistic goals first. Running into something unfamiliar might make you give up sooner than expected. A study has shown that illogical expectations and sudden changes in lifestyle are the usual reasons why individuals quit after 6 to 12 months. Which is why identifying your limits is important.

So before you plunge right into your diet, take some time to consider the following:

- What are your goals?
    - For your body measurements
    - For your daily nutritional needs
    - For your pre- and post-workout fuel
- Do you have a pre-existing condition?
    - Are you taking maintenance medicines?
    - What are the contraindications and special precautions of the medicines that you are taking?

- What are the nutritional requirements of your condition?
  - What are your anatomical and physiological genetic predispositions?
- Take a look at your family and identify similar physical characteristics.
- Take note of your family's physical activities. This will give you an idea of your physical strengths and weaknesses.
- What is your workout routine?
  - How often in a week can you do it?
  - What workout equipment is available to you?
- What is your lifestyle like?
  - Are you always eating out?
  - Are you always busy and don't have time to cook your meals?
  - Do you work from home and have enough time to prepare your meals?

Based on your answers, you can now devise a plan for how you can reach your goals. And determine how much macronutrients you will need to remain functional and healthy, while also burning excess calories.

Week 2: Replace Processed Food

As the saying goes, "Out of sight, out of mind."

Forget that they ever existed by removing everything that is processed or refined from your refrigerator and kitchen cabinet. And replace them with fresh produce.

It might help to create a grocery list before your trip to the supermarket. So that you can easily skip the aisles that contain processed and refined foods.

Examples of processed foods:

- Canned goods (except for sardines, tuna, salmon, and vegetables)
- Instant noodles
- Soft drinks and other flavored drinks
- Convenience foods:
    - Pizza
    - Granola
    - Energy bars
    - Breakfast cereal
    - Precooked foods
- Confections:
    - White and brown sugar
    - Corn and rice syrup
    - Candies
    - Dessert mixes
    - Sugar substitutes
    - Chocolate
    - Whipped cream
- Processed meat

- Sausage
- Ham
- Bacon
- Processed fats and oils:
    - Margarine
    - Salad dressing
    - BBQ sauce
    - Mayonnaise
    - Peanut butter

Week 3: Reduce Carbs

Carbs are easy to love because they relatively demand less time for cooking and eating, and they fill you up a lot faster. They also have cheaper options with a longer shelf life.

One study showed that consuming "fast-digesting" carbohydrates stimulates the nucleus accumbens in the brain, which plays a role in addictive behaviors. This is why frequent carbohydrate consumption is habit-forming and simple sugars are hard to limit in our diet.

So here are a few tips that you could follow to help you control carbohydrate consumption:

Step 1: Hydrate Yourself

Drink as much water as you can, especially two hours before meals. This makes you full faster and helps in controlling food cravings. Sometimes the urge to eat is just a signal that the body is dehydrated. So by drinking a lot of water, the craving can be suppressed.

Also, since limiting carbohydrates in the diet leads to difficulty in passing stool, hydration is important to keep your stool soft for an easy bowel movement.

Step 2: Snack Healthily

Whenever hunger pangs hit, make it a habit to munch on raw vegetables such as:

- Carrots
- Celery
- Frozen peas
- String beans
- Cucumbers
- Broccoli
- Cauliflower

And when a sugar craving kicks in, ask yourself first if a fruit will satisfy you. If the answer is yes, then what you are feeling is hunger. If not, then it is simply a craving.

Be sure to choose a fruit that does not contain too much sugar to avoid stimulating more of your cravings and to keep your insulin levels stable.

A few examples of fruits with 11 to 13 grams of sugar per serving:

- Lemons and limes
- Raspberries
- Strawberries
- Blackberries
- Kiwis
- Grapefruit
- Avocado
- Watermelon
- Cantaloupe
- Oranges
- Peaches

Step 3: Add Healthy Fats and Proteins

To keep up with the nutritional requirements of your body, you would have to take in a larger amount of healthy fats and protein.

By eating more protein, ghrelin (the hormone responsible for hunger) is decreased, your metabolic rate is increased after food intake and during rest, and your insulin levels become more stable.

Familiarize yourself with sources of healthy fats and proteins, and build a habit of substituting your carbs.

For example:

- Replace cereals with eggs
- Replace white bread with lettuce

- Replace pasta with spaghetti squash
- Replace candy with nuts, especially almonds

Week 4: Devise a Weekly Plan

For the Not-So-Busy

If you are the type who has a lot of free time to spare, you can opt for 5 small meals a day.

This technique encourages eating breakfast within one to two hours upon waking, and replenishing every three to four hours-- giving a total of 5 meals a day.

With this method, more effort is required for preparation. Perhaps, you can start planning your meals over the weekend so that you can save a lot of time during the weekdays.

The advantage of this technique is that you can control your hunger, keep insulin levels stable, and distribute nutrients evenly throughout the day.

Monday

Meal 1: Oats, cinnamon, sliced banana, raspberries, whey protein

Meal 2: Fruit salad with mango, kiwi, papaya, hard-boiled egg whites

Meal 3: Two sushi rolls with whole grain or wild rice, apple

Meal 4: Protein shake, banana, flaxseed oil

Meal 5: Lean steak, potato, salad, veggies

Tuesday

Meal 1: Muesli, mixed berries, protein shake

Meal 2: Grapes, egg whites

Meal 3: Chicken salad prepared with olive oil

Meal 4: Protein shake, canned salmon and dill on rye

Meal 5: Protein shake, prawns on a bed of veggies, brown rice

Wednesday

Meal 1: Egg white omelet, button mushrooms, diced tomato

Meal 2: Tuna, avocado, salad with lemon juice

Meal 3: Sliced turkey breasts, mixed salad, whole wheat pita

Meal 4: Beef jerky, orange

Meal 5: Protein shake, Chicken grilled asparagus, pepper, onion, celery, small baked potato

Thursday

Meal 1: Omelet, sliced tomato, sliced pepper, whole wheat bread, banana

Meal 2: Tuna and chickpea salad prepared with flaxseed oil

Meal 3: Shredded chicken, mashed avocado, olive oil and spinach on whole-grain crackers

Meal 4: Brown rice cake, protein shake

Meal 5: Protein shake, grilled salmon on a bed of greens, beans, peas, carrots, olive oil, lemon

Friday

Meal 1: Hard-boiled egg whites, whole wheat bread, fruit salad

Meal 2: Greek salad with chicken breast, flaxseed oil

Meal 3: Prawns and vegetables

Meal 4: Protein shake, diced banana, and walnuts

Meal 5: Protein shake, chicken mushrooms stuffed with feta, carrots, peas, and a small baked potato

Saturday

Meal 1: Oatmeal cinnamon, apple juice, whey protein (cooked together)

Meal 2: Protein shake, grapes, orange

Meal 3: Grilled cod, brown rice, mixed veggies

Meal 4: Protein shake, cantaloupe

Meal 5: Grilled chicken breasts, tomato relish wrapped in lettuce leaves

Sunday

Meal 1: Large flat mushrooms, baby leaf spinach, poached egg whites

Meal 2: Protein shake, carrots dipped in hummus, apple

Meal 3: Baked salmon fillet with spinach and leeks, brown rice

Meal 4: Protein shake, peach, mixed nuts

Meal 5: Chicken breast, small sweet potato, carrots, green veggies

For the Fitness Enthusiast

If you do strength training thrice a week, you can incorporate carb cycling and/or metabolic confusion into your endomorph diet. Wherein the number of carbohydrates will depend on your workout for the day. The heavier your workout, the larger your carbohydrate intake. This way, you can burn off what you eat.

Sample Diet

	Carbohydrate Consumption	**Grams of Carbs**
Monday: Strength	High	120 to 150 grams

Training		
Tuesday: Cardio Training	Low	50 to 75 grams
Wednesday: Strength Training	High	120 to 150 grams
Thursday: Cardio Training	Low	50 to 75 grams
Friday: Strength Training	High	120 to 150 grams
Saturday: Cardio Training	Low	50 to 75 grams
Sunday: Rest	Only healthy fats and protein	0 grams

You may make adjustments as you see fit.

Best Sources of Carbs

Samples of carbohydrates that you can include in your diet:

Sweet Potatoes: Rich in antioxidants, vitamins, and anti-inflammatory agents

Potatoes: They are easy to break down, increase satiety, and are rich in nutrients and vitamins.

Quinoa: Contains all nine essential amino acids, vitamins, and antioxidants.

Steel Cut Oats: Increases satiety but with a low glycemic index.

Black Beans: Good source of fiber with a low glycemic index.

Fruits: Packed with vitamins and antioxidants.

For the Busy Bee

If you lead a busy life, you can just stick to the basic endomorph diet and have the usual three meals a day. Keeping in mind the 30-35-35 rule.

Week 5: Find Ways to Sustain

Calorie-Counting Apps

Since calorie counting is crucial for an endomorph diet to be effective, it might help to download an app where you can watch your food consumption patterns and measure your daily caloric intake.

By logging your food intake, it will make you more accountable for the calories and nutrition of your food choices. In effect, aiding you in identifying your bad dietary habits.

Some of the calorie-counting apps are:

- My Fitness Pal
- Lose It!

- FatSecret
- Cron-o-meter
- SparkPeople

Serving Sizes or Portions

Once you start calorie-counting, you also need to familiarize yourself with the serving sizes or portions.

The serving size varies per food and can get confusing at the start. And gets trickier as you become more religious about it.

You will encounter measurements like *A watermelon provides 30 calories per 100 grams or 2/3 cup of watermelon cubes.*

Because of this, you would have to learn how to measure your food to log your calorie intake accurately. Hence, you would have to invest in a weighing scale and measuring cups.

Support Group

In the beginning, the spirit is still strong and soaring high. But towards the middle, when your motivation is starting to dwindle, you might need someone or a group of people to remind you of your goals.

There will also be a point, especially during your "withdrawal phase", where you will be experiencing all sorts of discomfort. Such as a sudden episode of dizziness, headache, or gastrointestinal symptoms. And when this happens, you will need people to help you get through this phase.

Sample Recipes

Here are a few recipes that you can try at home to inspire you. Once comfortable, you can now get creative and explore your ideas.

Chicken Breast (Baked)

Ingredients:

- 4 boneless, skinless chicken breasts
- 2 tablespoons olive oil
- 1 tablespoon dried thyme
- 1 tablespoon garlic powder
- 1 teaspoon kosher salt
- 1/2 teaspoon black pepper

Instructions:

1. Preheat the oven to 375 degrees F (190 degrees C).
2. Rinse the chicken breasts under cold water and pat dry with paper towels. Brush both sides of each breast with olive oil.
3. In a small bowl, mix together the thyme, garlic powder, kosher salt, and black pepper.
4. Sprinkle the seasoning mixture evenly over both sides of the chicken breasts.
5. Place the seasoned chicken breasts in a baking dish, making sure they are not touching.
6. Bake for 25-30 minutes, or until chicken is cooked through and no longer pink in the middle.
7. Let the chicken rest for 5 minutes before slicing and serving.

Grilled Chicken and Vegetables Skewers

Ingredients:

- 1 lb. boneless, skinless chicken breasts
- 1 medium zucchini, sliced
- 1 small red onion, cut into chunks
- 1 bell pepper, cut into chunks
- 2 tablespoons olive oil
- 1 teaspoon dried oregano
- 1 teaspoon garlic powder
- Salt and pepper to taste

Instructions:

1. Preheat grill to medium-high heat
2. Cut chicken into chunks and thread onto skewers alternating with zucchini, onion and pepper.
3. Drizzle olive oil over skewers and season with oregano, garlic powder, salt and pepper.
4. Grill skewers for 10-15 minutes, until chicken is cooked through and vegetables are charred.

Quinoa Salad with Avocado

Ingredients:

- 1 cup quinoa, cooked
- 1 avocado, diced
- 1 pint cherry tomatoes, halved
- 1 small red onion, diced
- 1 small bunch cilantro, chopped
- Juice of 1 lime
- 2 tablespoons olive oil
- Salt and pepper to taste

Instructions:

1. Combine cooked quinoa, avocado, cherry tomatoes, red onion, and cilantro in a bowl.
2. In a small bowl, whisk together lime juice, olive oil, salt and pepper.
3. Drizzle dressing over quinoa salad and toss to combine.

Baked Salmon with Sweet Potato Fries

Ingredients:

- 2 6-oz. salmon fillets
- 2 medium sweet potatoes, cut into fries
- 2 tablespoons olive oil
- 1 teaspoon smoked paprika
- 1 teaspoon garlic powder
- Salt and pepper to taste

Instructions:

1. Preheat oven to 400°F.
2. Toss sweet potato fries with olive oil, smoked paprika, garlic powder, and salt.
3. Spread fries out on a baking sheet and roast for 20-25 minutes, until crisp.
4. Season salmon fillets with salt and pepper and place on a separate baking sheet.
5. Roast salmon for 12-15 minutes, until cooked through.

Turkey Meatballs with Spaghetti Squash

Ingredients:

- 1 lb. ground turkey
- 1/2 cup almond flour
- 1 large egg
- 1/4 cup finely chopped basil
- 1 spaghetti squash, halved and seeded
- 2 tablespoons olive oil
- 1 teaspoon dried oregano
- 1 teaspoon garlic powder
- Salt and pepper to taste

Instructions:

1. Preheat oven to 375°F.
2. In a large bowl, combine ground turkey, almond flour, egg, basil, salt and pepper.
3. Form mixture into 12 evenly sized meatballs.
4. Drizzle olive oil over spaghetti squash and sprinkle with oregano, garlic powder, salt, and pepper.
5. Bake both meatballs and spaghetti squash for 20-25 minutes, until cooked through and tender.

Chicken and Broccoli Stir-Fry

Ingredients:

- 1 lb. boneless, skinless chicken breasts, sliced
- 1 head broccoli florets
- 2 carrots, sliced
- 1/4 cup soy sauce
- 2 tablespoons honey
- 1 tablespoon cornstarch
- 2 teaspoons ginger
- 1 garlic clove, minced
- 2 tablespoons olive oil
- Salt and pepper to taste

Instructions:

1. Heat olive oil in a wok over high heat.
2. Add chicken and stir-fry for 5-7 minutes, until cooked through.
3. Add broccoli and carrots to the wok and continue stir-frying for an additional 5-7 minutes.
4. In a small bowl, whisk together soy sauce, honey, cornstarch, ginger, garlic, salt and pepper.
5. Pour sauce over stir-fry and continue to cook for another 2-3 minutes, until sauce thickens.

Beef and Vegetable Stew

Ingredients:

- 1 lb. beef stew meat
- 1 large onion, chopped
- 2 garlic cloves, minced
- 4 cups low-sodium beef broth
- 1 cup sliced carrots
- 1 cup chopped celery
- 1 cup chopped sweet potato
- 1 cup sliced mushrooms
- 1/4 cup chopped parsley
- 2 tablespoons olive oil
- 1 teaspoon dried thyme
- Salt and pepper to taste

Instructions:

1. Heat olive oil in a large pot over medium-high heat.
2. Add stew meat and cook until browned on all sides.

Conclusion

Among the three body types, Endomorph is the most challenging in terms of staying in shape and remaining healthy due to its slow metabolism and inclination to convert more calories into stored fat. For men, being an endomorph is an advantage when it comes to strength sports and bodybuilding.

Fortunately, this genetic predisposition is not the end of the road. Lifestyle and diet can still be worked on to achieve a leaner physique.

One way of doing so is by taking advantage of their anatomical good points. Such as their great strength and propensity for muscle growth. Which could be maximized through strength training and high-intensity interval training.

The reduction in fat percentage and increase in muscle mass aid in the breakdown of fat during workouts and rest days.

Furthermore, coupling a good exercise program with an endomorph diet speeds up the transformation into a healthier endomorph body.

FAQ and Quick Summary

1. What is an endomorph?

An endomorph is a body type that is characterized by having a larger body size, higher levels of body fat, and a slower metabolism. This body type tends to store more fat around the midsection and lower body, which can make it harder to lose weight and maintain lean muscle mass.

2. What kind of diet should endomorphs follow?

Endomorphs should follow a balanced diet that focuses on quality protein sources, complex carbohydrates, and healthy fats. They should aim to eat mostly whole foods that are minimally processed and avoid highly processed foods that are high in added sugars, saturated fat, and sodium.

3. How much protein should endomorphs consume?

Endomorphs should aim to consume between 1.2–1.5 grams of protein per kilogram of body weight each day. This will help to support lean muscle mass and prevent muscle breakdown during weight loss.

4. What are some good sources of protein for endomorphs?

Good sources of protein for endomorphs include lean meats, poultry, fish, eggs, dairy products, and plant-based sources such as beans, lentils, and soy products.

5. What kind of complex carbohydrates should endomorphs consume?

Endomorphs should focus on consuming complex carbohydrates that are low in sugar and high in fiber. Good sources of complex carbohydrates include whole grains, vegetables, fruits, and legumes.

6. What kind of healthy fats should endomorphs consume?

Endomorphs should consume healthy fats that are high in omega-3 fatty acids such as fatty fish, flax seeds, chia seeds, and walnuts. Other good sources of healthy fats include olive oil, avocado, and nuts.

7. Should endomorphs count calories?

Endomorphs can benefit from tracking their calorie intake to ensure they are in a calorie deficit to lose weight. However, it is important to focus on the quality of the foods they are eating rather than just the number of calories.

8. What kind of exercise should endomorphs do?

Endomorphs should focus on both cardiovascular exercise and strength training. Cardiovascular exercise will help to burn calories, while strength training will help to build lean muscle mass and boost metabolism.

9. How often should endomorphs exercise?

Endomorphs should aim to exercise for at least 30 minutes a day, most days of the week. They should also incorporate at least two days of strength training each week.

10. How long does it take for endomorphs to see results?

Endomorphs can see results in as little as four to six weeks if they are following a balanced diet and exercise plan consistently. However, it is important to remember that weight loss is a gradual process and everyone's body responds differently.

References and Helpful Links

Sims, S. T., Ph.D. (2016, August 19). The 3 Body Types, Explained. Retrieved June 8, 2020, from https://www.runnersworld.com/health-injuries/a20818211/the-3-body-types-explained/

Drywień, M. E., Frąckiewicz, J., Górnicka, M., Ważna, B., Zielińska, P., Wójcik, K., & Kulik, S. (2017). Somatotype, diet, and nutritional status of women. Anthropological Review, 80(4), 393–404. https://doi.org/10.1515/anre-2017-0028

3 SOMATOTYPES. (n.d.). Retrieved June 8, 2020, from https://www.uh.edu/fitness/comm_educators/3_somatotypesNEW.htm

Drywień, M. E., Frąckiewicz, J., Górnicka, M., Ważna, B., Zielińska, P., Wójcik, K., & Kulik, S. (2017). Somatotype, diet and nutritional status of women. Anthropological Review, 80(4), 393–404. https://doi.org/10.1515/anre-2017-0028

THE 3 SOMATOTYPES. (n.d.). Retrieved June 8, 2020, from https://www.uh.edu/fitness/comm_educators/3_somatotypesNEW.htm

Sims, S. T., PhD. (2016, August 19). The 3 Body Types, Explained. Retrieved June 8, 2020, from https://www.runnersworld.com/health-injuries/a20818211/the-3-body-types-explained/

Huizen, J. (2019, June 27). What to know about the endomorph diet. Retrieved June 8, 2020, from https://www.medicalnewstoday.com/articles/325577#overview

Cellucor, T. (2018, February 1). Endomorph Diet & Workout Guide. Retrieved June 9, 2020, from https://c4energy.com/blogs/training/endomorph-diet-workout-guide

M. (2020, May 8). Metabolic Confusion for Endomorphs for Quick Fat Loss. Retrieved June 9, 2020, from https://www.libifit.com/metabolic-confusion-for-endomorphs/

Dalle Grave, R., Calugi, S., Molinari, E., Petroni, M. L., Bondi, M., Compare, A., & Marchesini, G. (2005). Weight Loss Expectations in Obese Patients and Treatment Attrition: An Observational Multicenter Study. Obesity Research, 13(11), 1961–1969. https://doi.org/10.1038/oby.2005.241

Bauer, S. M. (2020, March 25). What Is the Endomorph Diet and Could It Do More Harm Than Good? Retrieved June 9, 2020, from https://www.shape.com/healthy-eating/diet-tips/endomorph-diet

NPR Choice page. (2013, June 26). Retrieved June 17, 2020, from https://choice.npr.org/index.html?origin=https://www.npr.org/sections/thesalt/2013/06/26/195292850/can-you-be-addicted-to-carbs-scientists-are-checking-that-out#:%7E:text=Fast%2 Digesting%20 carbohydrates%20can%20 stimulate,pleasure%20 centers%20in%20the%20 brain.

Johnson, J. (2018, August 31). How do you manage food cravings? Retrieved June 14, 2020, from https://www.medicalnewstoday.com/articles/322947#mental-games

Cafasso, J. (2020, April 17). 11 Best Low-Sugar Fruits. Retrieved June 11, 2020, from https://www.healthline.com/health/best-low-sugar-fruits#lemons-and-limes

Spritzler, R. F. D. (2016, June 6). 14 Easy Ways to Increase Your Protein Intake. Retrieved June 11, 2020, from https://www.healthline.com/nutrition/14-ways-to-increase-protein-intake#section1

West, R. H. D. (2016, June 7). Counting Calories 101: How to Count Calories to Lose Weight. Retrieved June 11, 2020, from https://www.healthline.com/nutrition/counting-calories-101#section6

www.ingramcontent.com/pod-product-compliance
Lightning Source LLC
LaVergne TN
LVHW051925060526
838201LV00062B/4697